Lose Your Belly Diet

Incredible Healthy Recipes to Get Rid of That Annoying Belly

Table of Contents

Introduction

Congratulations on purchasing your personal copy of *Lose Your Belly Diet.* Thank you for doing so. You don't always need to exercise to lose weight, but it is always a good idea so you can remain in good physical condition.

Ask yourself a few important questions:

- Are you concerned about the extra weight you are carrying around your belly?
- Do you want to drop those pounds and still enjoy a tasty meal?

Of course, you do!

By purchasing your personal copy of *Lose Your Belly Diet,* you will be sure to have a healthy breakfast, lunch, or dinner meal fit to please even the choosiest of diners. Here are a few of the tasty menus to tempt your taste buds:

- Watermelon Paradise
- Wild Blueberry Soy Shake
- Hot Dish- Sausage Egg and Cheese
- Brownie Muffins
- Honey Mint Fruit Salad
- Greek Tuna Salad/Zesty Dressing
- Asian Tuna Patties
- Steelhead Trout Bake
- Apples and Cream Cheese Roll Ups
- Simmered Pears

You will know what to purchase and how to cook it with step by step instructions.

The recipes prepared for you in the following chapters are geared towards your satisfaction while at the same time providing you with lowered calorie content.

You will discover how important it is to pay attention to labels and the ways you can prepare everyday foods.

There are plenty of books on this subject on the market. Thanks again for choosing this one! Every effort was made to ensure it is full of as much useful information as possible. Please enjoy!

Index

Muffins

- Brownie Muffins
- Corn Apple Muffins
- Egg Muffins

Pancakes
- Blueberry Pancakes
- Cottage Cheese and Oatmeal Pancakes
- Hotcakes: Wheat-Free
- Skinny Pancakes

- Breakfast Cookies

Chapter 3: Lunch Favorites
- Bell Pepper Salad and Brown Rice
- Honey Mint Fruit Salad
- Tomato and Cucumber Salad

Poultry

- Chicken Manicotti and Spinach
- Chicken Salad / Low-Cal Mayonnaise
- Stuffed Turkey Burger

White Fish
- Cauliflower and Shrimp Salad
- Flounder – Spinach Stuffed with Mushrooms and Feta
- Greek Tuna Salad/Zesty Dressing
- Sole – Spinach Stuffed
- Spinach Sandwich and Tuna Salad
- Tuna and Broccoli
- Tuna Salad - Plain

Soups

- Celebration Chicken Soup
- Ginger Chicken Noodle Soup
- Gluten-Free Tortilla

Chapter 4: Dinner Favorites
Poultry

- Baked Chicken with Peppers and Mushrooms
- Blackened Chicken
- Chicken Cacciatore – Slow-Cooker
- Chicken Neapolitan
- Chicken Stir Fry
- Chicken Thighs with Turmeric
- Diet Cola Chicken
- Garlic Lime Chicken
- Indian Curry Chicken

White Fish

- Asian Tuna Patties
- Garlic Lemon Tilapia
- Marinated Tuna Steak – Grilled
- Microwave Tilapia
- Seared Sea Scallops
- Steelhead Trout Bake
- Szechwan Shrimp

Other Main Dishes
- Zucchini and Tomato Frittata
Sides and Veggies
- Beet Pesto Salad
- Cauliflower and Rice
- Mashed Cauliflower
- Potato Salad
- Zucchini Noodles

Chapter 5: Snacks and Appetizers

The Quick Fix Snacks
- By the Dish
- For Dipping
- Other Combos

Recipes for Snacks

- Bruschetta and Mint Pea Puree
- Jalapeno Fudge
- Mexican Jicama Snack

Sauces

- Hummus
- Italian Hummus
- Orange Basil Vinaigrette
- Salsa De Tomatillo
- Tzatziki Sauce
- Vegetable Salsa

Chapter 6: Desserts
- Apples and Cream Cheese Roll Ups
- Banana Bread (Whole Grain)
- Blueberry Shortbread Bites
- Coconut Chocolate Cookies
- Ginger Snap Cookies
- Simmered Pears
- Very Berry Tarts / Triple Berry Curd

Chapter 1: Ins and Outs of Weight Gain and Loss

To become successful at weight loss or gain takes practice. The following elements are just a few of the ways to get your eating habits back in line.

How Weight Loss and Weight Gain Works

You have to find and maintain a balance that works for you. What it comes down to, when you consider the bottom line – calories do count. Managing your weight is a balance of the number of calories you consume versus the amount that your body can effectively use up.

A calorie is a unit of energy which is delivered by food, no matter what the source. Whether you are consuming proteins, sugars, fats, or carbs – everything has a calorie count that needs to be considered.

To remain in balance, you must count the calories from your foods and balance it with your daily exercise and activity. This is how it works:

The Calorie Scale

You Weight Status	Your Calorie Status
Losing the weight	*Calorie deficit*: You will need to eat fewer calories than you are using. Your weight is decreasing because the fat storage cells are used for energy.
Gaining the weight	*Calorie excess*: Your body is not using the calories. They are stored as fat.
Maintaining the weight	*In balance*: You are stabilized with your weight by consuming the amount of calories you are using.

What to Eat

You are on the right path and need to be sure you are eating the right types of foods. These are some of the foods to place more focus on for your healthier habits:

- *Fresh, Canned, or Frozen Veggies*: You can use any of these items but consider using them without the additional sauces, butter, and extra salt. Try something new each week with seasonal items at the market.

- *Frozen, Fresh, or Canned Fruits*: Be creative on your choices in the fruit section, but remember to watch the calorie contents. Canned fruits may also have added syrups and sugars. Fresh is best, but be sure to read the labels if you purchase canned or frozen products.

- *Calcium-Rich Foods*: Enjoy some low-fat and fat-free yogurts without added sugars. You can make many different flavors. Some recipes for smoothies and shakes are in the breakfast section.

- *Alter the Methods of Cooking*: Consider using the grill, slow cooker, or oven instead of frying all of your foods. Your calorie counts will thank you.

The main thing to remember is to stay focused.

How to Snack Healthy

- *Always read the food panels.* You need to pay close attention for harmful additives. If you see a long list of ingredients that do not seem familiar, be aware.

- *Use pre-packaged snack packs.* Purchase items which already have the calorie counts for those times when you are in a rush and do not have time to prepare a healthy snack.

- *Precut fruits and veggies are best choices when you are watching your weight.* If your budget can handle a small increase, you will always be sure to have the right amount of calories for your food item.

- *Remove the temptations.* Losing belly fat is a much easier task if you are not constantly reminded by the food in the refrigerator and the pantry. Do a 'clean sweep' and remove the junk food. Donate it to a food bank or someone who is in need, if the products are unopened.

- *Plan ahead.* Make a lot of healthier snacks and place them in a Ziploc baggie for those times when you are hurrying out of the door.

- *Choose fiber food items.* While you are concentrating on losing weight, it is good to choose items with higher fiber content, so you have that 'full' feeling much longer.

Now, you have the idea. You are ready to begin your new healthier ways of eating to change your life!

Chapter 2: Breakfast Recipes

Smoothies and Shakes

Banana Rocket Smoothie

Ingredients
1 cup 1% fat milk
1 teaspoon each:
- Light brown sugar
- Vanilla extract

1 scoop vanilla soy protein powder
1 medium banana

Instructions
1. Add all of the goodies into a blender along with a couple of ice cubes.
2. Blend until smooth and drink right away. Don't wait more than 2 days because it will not be good.

Calories: 199
Yields: Two servings

Banana Mango Shake

Ingredients
1 small ripe sliced banana
½ ripe mango
½ cup each:
- Orange juice
- 1 % milk

1 tsp. sugar
2 tsp. each:
- Vanilla frozen yogurt - heaping
- Lime juice

Instructions
1. Peel and cut the outer skin away from the mango and add it to the blender in diced bits. Toss in the banana.
2. Add the remainder of the ingredients and blend about 30 seconds on the highest speed.
3. Pour into your glasses with some ice.
4. Garnish with some mango and mint if desired. (Add the additional calories.)

Calories: 150
Yields: Two servings

Banana Pear Smoothie

Ingredients
1 cup skim milk
1 teaspoon ginger root
2 ripe pears
1 banana
Sprinkle of cinnamon
1 handful of ice

Instructions
1. Pit and coarsely chop the ginger and pears.
2. Blend the ingredients and add a bit of cinnamon.

Calories: 199
Yields: Two servings

C-Blast Smoothie

Ingredients
1 large pink grapefruit
½ cup each:
- Non-fat Greek yogurt
- Strawberries

- Pineapple crushed/canned/fresh

Instructions
1. Peel, deseed, and cut the grapefruit into chunks.
2. Blend all of the fruits and yogurt.
3. Fresh or frozen – Add ¼ cup ice for froth

Calories: 159
Yields: Two servings

Citrus Energy-Enhancement

Ingredients
4 spinach leaves
2 carrots
1 each:
- Lemon
- Peach
- Orange

1 ½ - cups almond milk

Instructions
1. Peel, chop, and remove all skins and seeds from the fruit. Peel and chop/grate the carrots.
2. In a blender, combine all ingredients, and enjoy.

Calories: 143
Yields: Two servings

Easter Egg Fruity Delight – Smoothie

Ingredients
9 ice cubes - divided
9 tablespoons water -divided
9 tablespoons non-fat milk - divided
½ cup each of frozen:

- Blueberries
- Strawberries
- Pineapple

Instructions
1. Duplicate the process for each one.
2. Add 3 tablespoons of water, 3 tablespoons of milk, and 3 ice cubes along with the fruit in the blender.
3. Pour each of the prepared ingredients into a glass and place it in the freezer and move on until you finish the three units.
4. To serve, alternate the three tasty glasses into a serving glass/glasses, and enjoy.

Calories: 150
Yields: 2 Small or 1 large smoothie

Strawberry and Beet Smoothie

Ingredients
1 lime – juiced
2 cups each:
- Unsweetened coconut water
- Frozen strawberries
4 cooked and peeled beets

Instructions
1. Blend all of the goodies and enjoy!

Calories: 147
Yields: Two servings

Strawberry and Spinach Smoothie

Ingredients
2 cups fresh spinach

½ cup yogurt (low-fat vanilla)
1 cup sliced strawberries
2 cups water
1 medium banana
Optional: Maple syrup or honey

Instructions
1. Lightly pack and chop the spinach and add the remainder of ingredients to a blender.
2. Blend on the high setting and pour.

Calories: 120
Yields: Two servings

Strawberry Pineapple Smoothie

Ingredients
½ cup each:
- Halved strawberries
- Plain low-fat yogurt
- Pineapple juice

Optional: 1 banana

Instructions
1. Blend all of the ingredients until you like the consistency.

Calories: 138
Yields: Two servings

Watermelon Paradise

Ingredients
2 cups watermelon - chopped and seedless
1 cup each:
- Plain low-fat yogurt
- Strawberries

Handful of ice

Instructions
1. Blend the ingredients and enjoy.

Calories: 149
Yields: Two servings

Wild Blueberry Soy Shake

Ingredients
1 ½ - cups vanilla soy milk
4 tablespoons honey
2 cups frozen wild blueberries
1 dash each:
- Freshly ground nutmeg
- Fresh mint leaves

Instructions
1. Combine the milk, honey, and frozen berries in a blender.
2. Puree until creamy smooth and add your garnishes if desired.

Calories: 140 each
Yields: Four servings

Eggs
Baked Egg Cups

6 eggs
6 slices lean deli ham
½ cup cheddar cheese (2% shredded)
1 tablespoon chopped chives
Pepper

Instructions

1. Set the oven to 350°F. Prepare a muffin tin using the cooking spray. Place the slices of ham into six cups, so it is completely covered with the edges of ham above the cup.
2. Bake 10 minutes, remove and add one broken egg to each cup. Pepper if desired and cook ten more minutes.
3. When the egg is to your desired doneness, remove and sprinkle with cheese and chives. Serve immediately.

Calories: 125.6 each
Yields: Six servings

Broccoli, Mushroom, and Sausage Quiche

Ingredients
12 ounces turkey sausage
1 cup broccoli (chopped)
6 medium mushrooms (sliced)
6 egg whites
¼ cup each:
- Flour
- Colby cheese (shredded)
- Cottage cheese (2%)
1 cup soy milk
1 teaspoon garlic (minced)

Instructions

1. Set the oven at 350°F. Spray a nine-inch baking pan with some cooking oil.
2. Prepare the sausage in a skillet and crumble. Put to the side.
3. Blend the cheeses, egg whites, flour, milk, and garlic.
4. Combine and add the sausage, broccoli, and sausage into the pan.
5. Your quiche will be ready in 30 minutes.

Calories: 142
Yields: Eight servings

Canadian Bacon and Chicken Quiche

Ingredients
4 large eggs
1 small sweet red and 1 green bell pepper (diced)
½ cup skim milk
¼ cup sharp cheddar cheese
1 cup chicken (diced)
3 ounces Canadian bacon (diced)

Instructions
1. Preheat the oven to 325°F.
2. Combine the eggs, milk, cheese, chicken (cooked), bacon, sweet and green peppers.
3. Mix well and pour the batter into a round baking dish and bake for approximately 25 minutes.

Calories: 193
Yields: Four servings

Chicken and Egg Muffins/Buffalo Style

Ingredients
6 ounces chicken (chopped and cooked)
8 eggs
2 ½ tablespoons buffalo wing sauce
1/8 cup blue cheese (crumbled)
1 chopped rib of celery
2 chopped green onions
1 minced clove of garlic
Optional:
- Sea salt
- Pepper

Instructions

1. Oven setting: 350°F. Grease/oil the muffin pan.
2. Use a fork to whip the eggs. Mix all ingredients thoroughly and place in the tins.
3. Bake until fluffy—about 20 minutes.

Calories: 200
Yields: 8 muffins (Four servings)

Deviled Eggs

6 hard-boiled eggs
¼ teaspoon each:
- Black Pepper
- Salt

½ teaspoon dry mustard
2 tablespoons mayonnaise

Instructions

1. Prepare the eggs by slicing them lengthwise in halves.
2. Mash the yolks in a separate dish—add mustard—mayonnaise—pepper—and salt.
3. Fill the whites with the mixture and serve.

Calories: 84 (50 g)
Yields: Each serving is 50 g

Eggs and Bacon

Ingredients
3 ½ ounces full-fat cream cheese
6 extra-large hard-boiled organic eggs
¼ teaspoon dried organic thyme

Instructions
1. Set the oven at 400°F.

2. Mix the thyme and cream cheese.
3. Peel the eggs and slice them with a sharp knife, lengthwise.
4. Dump the egg yolks into a dish and mix with the remainder of the ingredients.
5. Fill the eggs with the mixture.
6. For each egg, begin by wrapping the bacon tightly around each one.
7. Bake for 30 minutes in a casserole dish.

Calories: 200
Yields: 12 servings

Egg Clouds

Ingredients
4 large eggs
¼ cup chopped chives
¼ cup parmesan cheese (shredded)
3 bacon strips
Optional: Pepper

Instructions
1. Preheat the oven at 450°F.
2. Use four separate bowls. Separate the eggs by putting the whites in one, yolks, in another, shells in a bowl for the trash, and one for mixing the ingredients.
3. Whip/Whisk the whites to form stiff peaks using a metal mixing container. (A blender or electric mixer will be sufficient.)
4. Slowly, fold in the bacon, chives, and cheese.
5. Use parchment paper to line the baking sheet. Spoon four mounds of stiff egg whites onto the sheet. Make a well in the center of each of the mounds.
6. Bake for three minutes, and remove it from the oven.

7. Add one yolk to each cloud and season it to your taste. Bake about two or three more minutes for a soft yolk.

Calories: 161 each
Yields: Four servings

Egg Whites and Tomatoes

Ingredients
2 egg whites
¼ cup diced tomato

Instructions
1. Combine the ingredients.
2. Fry together on medium heat.

Calories: 41
Yields: One serving

Hot Dish – Sausage Egg and Cheese

Ingredients
½ pound ground pork
10 medium eggs
6 bread slices
1 ½ - cups milk
1/8 teaspoon mustard
4 ounces cheddar cheese (shredded)
½ teaspoon each:
   - Salt
   - Pepper

Instructions
1. Cook the sausage normally.
2. Toast the bread on a lightly greased baking dish (9 x 13 is a good size).

3. Scramble the eggs and mix with the milk.
4. Add the mustard, salt, and pepper as you like it.
5. Add the crumbled sausage and mix.
6. Pour the mixture over the toast.
7. Add the cheese and let it set overnight.
8. The next morning, bake at 350°F.
9. Bake the prepared dish for 25 minutes or until done.

Calories: 151
Yields: 12 Servings

Quiche Cups

Ingredients
2 cups frozen spinach (chopped)
½ onion (sliced)
2 cups egg beaters®
½ cup mozzarella cheese (shredded)
½ teaspoon hot sauce

Instructions
1. Microwave the onion and spinach until the onion is soft, and the spinach is thawed.
2. Combine everything and flavor with pepper and salt.
3. Bake at 375°F for 20 minutes using a muffin tin.

Calories: 105 each (112.7 grams each serving)
Yields: Approximately four servings

Southwestern Chicken Fajita Quiche

Ingredients
1 package McCormick Taco Seasoning Mix (gluten-free)
24 large egg whites
12 ounces grilled chicken breast (diced)
2 medium bell peppers (steamed and diced)

Instructions

1. Preheat the oven at 300F.
2. Spray non-stick cooking oil onto (2) nine-inch round baking pans.
3. Whisk the taco mix and egg whites. Add the peppers and chicken.
4. Prepare in the oven approximately 25 to 30 minutes or when the center no longer jiggles. Leave the quiche in the pan for ten or fifteen minutes before serving.

Calories: 128 (2 slices)
Yields: 16 slices

Veggie Omelet – Slow Cooker

Ingredients
8 eggs
¼ tsp. each:
- Pepper
- Salt

1 tbsp. olive oil
½ cup each:
- Parmesan cheese - grated
- Potatoes
- Carrots
- Diced zucchini

1 medium onion
¼ cup each:
- Diced red bell peppers
- String/green beans – discarded ends

Instructions

1. Peel and dice the carrots and potatoes. Coarsely chop the green beans and onion. Whisk the eggs, pepper, salt, and parmesan cheese.

2. Add the oil (extra-virgin) into a pan. Saute the onions for two minutes (medium heat setting) before adding the rest of the veggies. Cook ten more minutes.
3. Dump the veggies into the slow cooker and add the egg mixture. (Be sure the veggies are covered.)
4. Cook on high for two hours

Calories: 167
Yields: Six servings

Muffins
Brownie Muffins

Ingredients
½ teaspoon salt
¼ cup cocoa powder
½ tbsp. baking powder
1 cup flaxseed meal
1 tbsp. cinnamon
½ cup pumpkin puree
2 tbsp. coconut oil
1 large egg
¼ cup sugar-free caramel syrup
1 teaspoon each:
   ▪ Apple cider vinegar
   ▪ Vanilla extract

Instructions
1. Set the oven temperature at 350°F.
2. In a deep bowl, mix each of ingredients.
3. Use six paper liners in the muffin tin, and add ¼ cup batter to each one.
4. Sprinkle a pinch of coconut on the tops.
5. Bake approximately 15 minutes when the top is set.

Calories: 182 (1 muffin each serving)

Corn Apple Muffins

Ingredients
1 tbsp. baking powder
½ cup yellow corn meal
¼ cup brown sugar
2 cup all-purpose flour
¼ tsp. salt
2 egg whites
1 apple
½ cup corn kernels
¾ cup fat-free milk

Instructions
1. Peel and coarsely chop the apple. Pack the brown sugar in the cup tightly.
2. Use a 12 count muffin pan and line the containers with foil or paper liners.
3. Program the oven temperature to 425°F.
4. Combine the brown sugar, cornmeal, salt, flour, and baking powder completely in a large mixing container.
5. Using a separate mixing container whip the egg whites and milk. Blend in the corn kernels along with the apple bits.
6. Whisk again and pour the batter into the flour mixture. Continue to gently stir the ingredients until slightly moistened.
7. Fill the cups 2/3 full. Bake for approximately thirty minutes.
8. Test the muffins for doneness by gently pressing the center. They should spring back.

Calories: 120 each
Yields: 12 muffins

Egg Muffins

Ingredients
1 tbsp. olive oil
6 eggs
2 cups fresh spinach
¼ diced cut onion
1 garlic clove
¾ cup cheddar cheese (shredded reduced-fat)
3 slices turkey bacon (chopped and cooked)
1 tablespoon milk
½ teaspoon each:
- Black Pepper
- Salt

Instructions
1. Place the oven setting at 350°F. Prepare a sauté pan using the oil.
2. Combine the onion and prepare them on the medium setting for approximately two minutes. Blend the spinach with the onions until it wilts in two or three more minutes.
3. Toss the garlic in the pan and continue cooking for 30 seconds. Spice it with pepper and salt.
4. Whip the milk, cheese, and eggs in a separate dish. Pitch in the bacon and spinach mixture.
5. Fill the muffin tins about ¾ full. Bake until they are lightly browned around the edges (about 20 minutes).

Note: Reheat them for 20 to 30 seconds in the microwave.

Calories: 148.6
Yields: Five servings

Pancakes

Blueberry Pancakes

Ingredients
2 large eggs
3 ounces milk (6 tablespoons)
2 tbsp. sugar
Pinch of salt
1 cup flour
1 tsp. baking powder
1 cup blueberries

Instructions
1. Empty the milk and add the egg yolks into a large mixing dish.
2. Sift in the flour, salt, and sugar to mix well.
3. Whip the egg whites into stiff peaks and blend into the flour mix. Blend in the berries.
4. Drop the mixture into the pan and cook until the bottom is browned, flip and finish cooking.
5. Top with your favorite topping, but count the extra calories.

Calories: 139
Yields: Six servings

Cottage Cheese and Oatmeal Pancakes

Ingredients
4 egg whites
½ cup cottage cheese (fat-free)
½ teaspoon each:
  ▪ Vanilla
  ▪ Baking powder
1 packet Stevia (2 for sweeter pancakes)

½ cup dry oatmeal

Instructions
1. Use a blender, and mix everything except for the oats.
2. Gradually add the oats because you want the mixture/batter lumpy.
3. Note: If you add berries; add after it is blended.
4. Cook over medium heat.
5. Top with your favorite topping.

Calories: 47.5
Yields: Six servings

Hotcakes: Wheat-Free

Ingredients
3 cups almond meal
1 tablespoon flaxseed (ground)
½ teaspoon each:
- Sea salt
- Baking soda

¾ cup regular/light coconut/almond milk
3 large eggs
2 tablespoons coconut oil/ melted butter/extra-light olive oil

Instructions
1. Combine the dry ingredients dish.
2. Use a whisk to mix the eggs, milk, and oil.
3. Use medium heat to prepare the pan with a small amount of oil.
4. Pour ¼ of the mixture into the skillet and cook for three minutes. Continue the process until done.

Calories: 162
Yields: 14 - Four-inch pancakes

Skinny Pancakes

Ingredients
¼ cup egg whites
1/3 tablespoon baking powder
½ teaspoon vanilla

Instructions
1. Mix all of the ingredients until it looks fluffy in the bowl.
2. Spray the skillet with some non-stick spray.
3. Lightly toast the pancakes until brown.

Total Calories: 43
Yields: One serving

Breakfast Cookies

Ingredients
1 cup quick oats
2 bananas
1 teaspoon cinnamon

Instructions
1. Set the oven temperature in advance to 350°F. Prepare a baking pan/sheet with a small amount of oil or some cooking spray.
2. Smash the bananas and stir in the oats. Toss in the cinnamon and stir.
3. Use a tablespoon to drop them onto the prepared sheet, and bake for fifteen minutes.

Calories: 50 (1 cookie)
Yields: 12 cookies

Chapter 3: Lunch Favorites

Bell Pepper Salad and Brown Rice

Ingredients
½ cup each diced red, yellow and green pepper
4 cups rice (cooked and brown)
1 chopped jalapeno
1 cup each:
- Black beans
- Diced tomatoes

1 bunch chopped cilantro
¾ cup spicy brown mustard
1 cup light mayo
5 ounces chopped sweet onion
¼ teaspoon chili powder

Instructions
1. Rinse and drain the black beans.
2. Chop the tops and bottoms from each of the peppers. Remove the seeds and dice them up. Add the beans, rice, tomato and onions.
3. In another dish combine the pepper, salt, chili powder, mayo, and brown mustard. Pour it over the pepper/rice mixture until covered.
4. Toss in the cilantro and gently mix.
5. Refrigerate overnight if possible or a minimum of several hours.

Calories: 163
Yields: 12 servings

Honey Mint Fruit Salad

Ingredients
1 fresh peach

¼ cup each:
- Honeydew melon – sliced
- Fresh blueberries
- Fresh sliced strawberries

1 tablespoon each:
- Honey
- Lime juice

2 tablespoons chopped fresh mint

Instructions
1. Toss all of the fruit in the serving dishes and top off with the lime juice.
2. Sprinkle some honey and a bit of mint.

Calories: 92 (1 cup)
Yields Two servings

Poultry
Chicken Manicotti and Spinach

Ingredients
1 cup chicken breast
2 cups spinach
2 ounces manicotti pasta
1 ½ cups spaghetti sauce
3 tablespoons pepper
2 teaspoons ground oregano
2 tablespoons garlic powder
½ cup water
¼ cup fat-free ricotta cheese
½ cup marble cheese
Optional: Chili powder

Instructions
1. Program oven temperature to 350°F.

2. Cook and dice the chicken. Prepare the pasta for about 6 minutes.
3. Combine the spinach, chicken, ricotta cheese, spices, and chili powder (if using).
4. Drain and cool the pasta, laying them out over the countertop to avoid getting stuck together. Stuff each of the noodles, blocking one end with your finger.
5. Arrange them in rows in a greased cooking pan and cover with the sauce. Pour the water into the dish with the sauce, and cover with some aluminum foil.
6. Bake 25 minutes, remove the foil and sprinkle with cheese.
7. Complement the meal with some steamed veggies or a side salad, but don't forget to add the additional calories.

Calories: 117 per serving
Yields: Ten servings

Chicken Salad

Ingredients
¼ cup each:
- Diced celery
- Green pepper

½ cup cooked green peas
4 lettuce leaves
2 stuffed olives - finely chopped
Pepper and salt to taste
8 tbsp. low-cal. mayo (recipe below)
1 cup cooked - diced chicken

Instructions
1. Thoroughly combine all of the ingredients (omit lettuce) in a salad dish. Blend in the mayo and toss.
2. Serve on the leaves of lettuce.

Calories: 89
Yields: Four servings

Low-Cal Mayonnaise

Ingredients
1 egg yolk
Pinch cayenne pepper
¼ teaspoon each:
- Salt
- Paprika

½ teaspoon dry mustard
1 drop liquid sweetener
¾ cup plain yogurt
1 tablespoon cider vinegar

Instructions
1. Beat the egg yolk and add in the rest of the ingredients. Chill.

Stuffed Turkey Burger

Ingredients
1 cup seasoned stuffing mix
½ cup chicken broth
1 teaspoon garlic powder
¼ cup barbecue sauce
12 ounces lean ground turkey

Instructions
1. Combine the stuffing with the broth and stir well. Let the mixture soften for five to six minutes.
2. Combine the garlic powder, barbecue sauce, wet stuffing, and ground turkey. Add to a bowl. Divide the mixture into four equal sections.
3. Grill or pan-fry and enjoy.

Calories: 177
Yields: Four servings

White Fish
Cauliflower and Shrimp Salad

Ingredients
1 pound raw shrimp (medium)
1 head of cauliflower
2 cucumbers
1 tablespoon and ¼ c. olive oil
3 tablespoons fresh dill (chopped)
2 tablespoons lemon zest (grated)
¼ cup fresh lemon juice

Instructions
1. Peel, clean, and remove the tail from the shrimp. Place them on a baking tin. Sprinkle them with the olive oil.
2. Roast at 350°F approximately 8 to 10 minutes (remove when opaque).
3. Chop the cauliflower into small pieces (trash the head).
4. Microwave the florets in a shallow bowl for 5 minutes until it has a soft texture (not mushy). Let it cool.
5. Peel, remove the seed and chop the cucumbers into ½ inch pieces.
6. After the shrimp have cooled, slice them lengthwise or chop them up.
7. Combine the cucumber, cauliflower, and the shrimp. Add the chopped dill and lemon zest.

Note: Hold the ¼ cup lemon juice or the remainder of the olive oil (1/4 cup) mixture that can be used as a dressing.

Calories: 200 (1 cup)
Yield: Six cups

Flounder – Spinach Stuffed with Mushrooms and Feta

Ingredients
8 ounces spinach
8 large mushrooms
4 (4 ounces) fillets of flounder
1 tablespoon crumbled feta cheese

Instructions
1. Rinse and chop the spinach and slice the mushrooms.
2. Preheat the oven to 350°F.
3. Coat a skillet with some non-stick cooking spray. Use the medium setting and sauté the mushrooms for five minutes.
4. Toss in the spinach and continue sautéing for approximately two minutes. Once the spinach wilts, transfer it to a plate and drain the moisture. Sprinkle the cheese over the veggies and stir.
5. *Assemble the Fish Rolls:* On the wide end of the fillet, add the spinach mix and roll it. Secure the roll with toothpicks.
6. Spray a baking dish (8x8) with the cooking oil. Arrange the fish rolls with the seam down into the dish.
7. Add two tablespoons of water and loosely cover the dish with some foil.
8. Bake in the hot oven until it is flaky or for about 15 to 20 minutes.

Calories: 131
Yields: Four servings

Greek Tuna Salad

Ingredients
1 (18 ounces) chunk light tuna (packed in water)
6 ounces pepperoncini (drained and sliced)

9 cups romaine lettuce

2 cups cucumber (peel on/diced)

1 cup cherry tomatoes (halved)

¾ cup each:

- Feta cheese crumbles (reduced fat)
- Red onion (rings)

18 black olives (sliced)

Zesty Dressing (Optional)

1 ½ - tsp. oregano

¼ cup olive oil

½ tsp. black pepper

2 tbsp. red wine vinegar

½ teaspoon salt – to taste

Instructions

1. Mix all ingredients for the salad (first list).
2. Mix all ingredients for the dressing (optional).
3. *Note*: Dressing not calculated in nutrition counts

Calories: 169

Yields: Six servings

Sole—Spinach Stuffed

Ingredients

2 cups fresh spinach leaves

1 teaspoon olive oil

Ground black pepper

2 teaspoons minced garlic

½ teaspoon melted butter

2 (5 ounces) sole/flounder fillets

Instructions

1. Lightly spray a coat of a nonstick cooking spray to a baking pan/dish.
2. Set the oven temperature to 400°F.
3. Use the stovetop and set the burner to a medium heat setting. Heat the oil and toss in the pepper, spinach, and garlic. Sauté about two or three minutes or until the spinach begins to wilt.
4. Put the fillets on the prepared baking dish. Put half of the mixture of spinach in the center of each fillet and roll them up.
5. Put them into the pan with the seam side down, brushing with the butter.
6. Bake about eight to ten minutes until the fish is opaque.

Calories: 157
Yields: Two servings

Spinach Sandwich and Tuna Salad

Ingredients
1 pouch (64 ounces) light tuna packaged in water
½ small red onion (about 1/4 cup peeled and diced)
½ medium cucumber
½ teaspoon each:
  ▪ Dill weed
  ▪ Salt-free seasoning blend
2 diced ribs of celery
1/4 teaspoon black pepper
Juice of one lemon
8 slices- (100%) whole wheat bread
2 tablespoons olive oil
1 cup fresh baby spinach leaves

Instructions

1. Peel, deseed, and dice the cucumber.
2. Mix the tuna, onion, cucumber, dill weed, and celery. Lightly drizzle the olive oil and lemon juice. Stir.
3. Use the pepper and seasoning blend to flavor the mixture.
4. Make the sandwich using ¼ of the spinach leaves and ½ cup of the tuna salad. (You can keep the tuna in the refrigerator for three days.)

Calories: 194
Yields: Two cups of tuna: Four servings

Tuna and Broccoli

Ingredients
1 can (3 ounces) light tuna
1 cup broccoli
2 tablespoons cheese
1 teaspoon salt

Instructions

1. Place the frozen florets of broccoli into the water until they are thawed, and drain.
2. Mix the broccoli and the cheese until melted.
3. Add the tuna. Salt if desired.

Calories: 122
Yields: Two servings

Tuna Salad – Plain

Ingredients
12 ounces canned tuna
½ cup Miracle Whip (fat-free)
4 green onions
3 eggs (hard-boiled)

1 tablespoon sweet pickle
Whole-wheat bread

Instructions
1. Mix all of the ingredients.
2. Put on whole wheat bread.

Calories: 165 (1/4 cup serving)
Yields: Eight servings

Soups

Celebration Chicken Soup – Slow Cooker

Ingredients

2 chicken breast fillets

1 minced garlic clove

½ cup diced onion

2 ½ cups chicken broth

1 can each (15 oz.):

- Black beans
- Kidney beans

1 can each:

- 14 ½ oz. diced tomatoes
- 4 ½ oz. green diced chili peppers

1 cup frozen or fresh corn

1 lime – juice

1 tbsp. chili powder

½ teaspoon each:

- Black pepper
- Cayenne pepper

Sea/kosher salt if desired

1 teaspoon cumin

½ cup freshly chopped cilantro

Instructions

1. Use the fat-free -low-sodium broth for this calorie count.
2. Cut the chicken into ½-inch cubes. Add all of the ingredients. Don't precook, but be sure to remove all skin.
3. Cook on the low setting (lid on) for six to eight hours.

Calories: 192 (1 cup portion)

Yields: 10 cups/servings

Ginger Chicken Noodle Soup

Ingredients

1 tbsp. olive oil

3 ounces dried soba noodles
1 large chopped yellow onion
1 carrot
1 clove of garlic
1 tbsp. fresh ginger
2 tbsp. soy sauce (reduced-sodium)
4 cups chicken broth or stock
1 cup shelled Edamame
1 pound chopped chicken breasts (no skin or bones)
¼ cup fresh chopped cilantro/coriander
1 cup plain soya/soy milk

Instructions
1. Mince the ginger and garlic clove. Peel and chop the carrot.
2. Bring the noodles to a boil in a pot about ¾ full of boiling water for five minutes.
3. Use the stovetop and set the burner to medium heat. Heat the oil and sauté the onion approximately four minutes.
4. Toss in the carrot and ginger and sauté one more minute. Then, add the garlic - sautéing for another thirty seconds (don't brown the garlic).
5. Pour the soy sauce and add the Edamame and chicken. When it starts to boil, lower the burner to the med-low setting. Cook about four more minutes.
6. Add the soy milk and noodles, cooking until completely heated.
7. Remove the skillet from the burner and toss in the cilantro.
8. Scoop into serving dishes and enjoy.

Calories: 184
Yields: Eight servings

Gluten-Free Tortillas

Ingredients
1 tablespoon coconut flour
½ teaspoon salt
½ cup (plus) 2 tablespoons dark flax meal
1 teaspoon olive oil
1/8 teaspoon chili powder
3 tablespoons hot water

Instructions
1. Combine the coconut flour, ½ cup of the flax meal, the chili powder, and salt. Set them to the side.
2. In a separate container, mix the oil, hot water, and the remainder of the flax meal. Combine the ingredients and mix thoroughly.
3. With gloved hands knead the dough around five minutes until it is creamy smooth. Divide them into four pieces.
4. Roll out the dough until flattened between two pieces of waxed or parchment paper. You can use a rolling pin or an empty wine bottle or glass.
5. Over med-high heat, cook the tortillas in a 10-inch skillet one at a time. Cook one minute and flip cooking until the tortilla slightly puffy.

Calories: 120
Yields: Four servings

Chapter 4: Dinner Favorites

Poultry

Baked Chicken with Peppers and Mushrooms
Ingredients
2 ½ cups sliced mushrooms
1 pound chicken breasts
1 tablespoon minced onion flakes
¼ cup soy sauce
2 tablespoons clover honey
½ cup chopped red pepper
1 teaspoon garlic powder

Instructions
1. Program the oven to 350°F. Arrange the chicken in a dish (9x13).
2. Shake the flakes of onion over the breasts.
3. In another container, mix the soy sauce, garlic powder, and honey. Empty that over the chicken.
4. Place a top on the baking dish for 30 minutes.
5. Add the green/red peppers to the dish and continue baking for 20 additional minutes with the dish covered. It is ready when the mushrooms are tender.

Calories: 179
Yields: Four servings

Blackened Chicken

Ingredients
¼ teaspoon each:
- Cayenne pepper
- Ground cumin
- Dried thyme

½ teaspoon paprika

1/8 teaspoon each:
- Salt
- Ground white pepper
- Onion powder

2 chicken breast halves (boneless and skinless)

Instructions
1. Set the oven temperature in advance to 350ºF. Grease a baking dish with some cooking spray or use aluminum foil for easier cleanup.
2. Use a cast iron skillet, and warm it on high for about five minutes.
3. Combine the onion powder, salt, paprika, thyme, cumin, cayenne, and white pepper.
4. Lightly spray each of the breasts and cover with the spice mix.
5. Add the chicken to the scalding skillet for one minute. Flip it over and cook for one more minute.
6. Arrange the breasts on the baking dish and bake about five minutes. The center juices should run clear when the chicken is done.

Calories: 135
Yields: Two servings

Chicken Cacciatore - Slow-Cooker

Ingredients
3 whole chicken breasts halved skinless
Dash of pepper
1 teaspoon salt
1 finely chopped green pepper
1 tablespoon dry onion flakes
1 minced garlic clove
2 teaspoons tomato paste

1 can each:
- 15 ounces diced tomatoes
- 4 ounces sliced - drained mushrooms

1 bay leaf
2 tablespoons chopped pimiento
¼ teaspoon thyme

Instructions
1. Wash and pat dry the chicken.
2. Mix all of the ingredients in the slow cooker making sure to thoroughly cover the chicken.
3. Place the lid on the cooker for seven to eight hours.

Calories: 120
Yields: Six servings

Chicken Neapolitan

Ingredients
2 medium chicken breasts (halved- no bones or skin)
2 tablespoons grated parmesan cheese
4 tablespoons each:
- Reduced-calorie Italian dressing - bottled
- Flavored dried breadcrumbs

1 teaspoon paprika
1 tablespoon sesame seeds

Instructions
1. Set the oven temperature to 400°F.
2. Use some spray cooking oil in a 12x8 baking dish.
3. Blend the cheese, breadcrumbs, cheese, paprika, and sesame seeds.
4. Dip each of the breasts in the dressing and coat them with the crumbs.
5. Place the breasts in the baking dish for about twenty minutes. Flip and bake an additional twenty minutes.

Calories: 100 each
Yields: Four servings

Chicken Stir Fry

Ingredients
1 lb. chicken breasts
¼ cup chicken stock
2 cups slices/pieces mushrooms
1 medium carrot
 1 cup each:
- Asparagus
- Chopped broccoli florets

¼ teaspoon cayenne pepper
1 teaspoon ginger
1 large egg

Instructions
1. Use the stovetop (medium-high heat) or a wok to warm the chicken stock.

Calories: 168
Yields: Four servings

Chicken Thighs with Turmeric

Ingredients
2 skinless, boneless chicken thighs
1 (one-inch) piece turmeric root
½ teaspoon sea salt
1 ½ teaspoons vegetable oil
Also Needed: Mortar and pestle

Instructions
1. Use the mortar and pestle to grind the sea salt and turmeric. Rub it over the thighs. Cover for about an hour using some plastic wrap.
2. Warm up the oil over medium heat and cook the chicken for about eight minutes. Flip and continue another eight minutes or until an internal thermometer reads 165°F.

Calories: 187
Yields: Two servings

Diet Cola Chicken

Ingredients
1 pound chicken breast meat
1 can diet soda
1 cup ketchup

Instructions
1. Combine the cola and ketchup.
2. Place the breasts in a skillet and add the cola/ketchup combination over the top and sides.
3. Cook the chicken over medium heat for about thirty minutes.
4. Remove the top. Cook for approximately ten to fifteen minutes more until the sauce begins sticking to the chicken.

Calories: 184 per serving
Yields: Four servings

Garlic Lime Chicken

Ingredients
1 pound chicken breasts – skinless – boneless
2 teaspoons minced garlic
½ teaspoon each:
- Dried mustard
- Ground black pepper

¼ cup fresh lime juice
½ cup soy sauce
Worcestershire sauce

Instructions
1. In a re-closable Ziploc-type bag, mix all of the ingredients for the marinade. Add the breasts and close the bag.
2. Toss the mixture and let it marinate in the fridge for a minimum of two hours.
3. When done, drain the juices, and grill/broil. Garnish as desired

Calories: 147 each
Yields: Four servings

Indian Curry Chicken

Ingredients
¼ cup Italian non-fat dressing
1 cup chopped onion
¼ teaspoon turmeric
3 teaspoons fresh ginger
½ teaspoon each:
- Curry powder
- Crushed red pepper

2 chicken breasts – skinless
½ cup chicken broth
1 tablespoon olive oil

Pinch of pepper and salt

Instructions

1. Add the Italian dressing, curry powder, turmeric, red pepper, ginger, and onion into an 8x8x2-inch glass baking dish.
2. Arrange the chicken in the marinade, cover, and stash it in the fridge for a minimum of two hours or one day.
3. Remove the chicken - saving the marinade. Pat it dry and season it with the pepper and salt.
4. Add oil to a skillet using the med-high setting. Arrange the chicken in the pan and saute until done (around three minutes for each side).
5. Blend the broth and marinade until it boils. Lower the heat setting to med-low and continue cooking for another six minutes.

Calories: 191 each serving
Yields: Four servings

White Fish
Asian Tuna Patties
Ingredients
2 cans light tuna/drained
1 teaspoon sesame oil
2 slices bread (wheat reduced-calorie or ¾ cup dry breadcrumbs)
¼ cup egg substitute (Eggbeaters is good)
1 clove garlic (peeled and minced)
3 green onions (minced)
1 teaspoon black pepper
1 tablespoon each of teriyaki sauce—ketchup—soy sauce
Non-stick cooking spray

Instructions
1. *For the Breadcrumbs:* Bake the slices at 200°F until they are crispy. Put them in a blender or food processor to equal ¾ cup.
2. Mix the egg, tuna, bread crumbs, garlic, and green onions in a large bowl.
3. Blend the teriyaki sauce, soy sauce, ketchup, pepper, and sesame oil into the mixture.
4. Shape the tuna patties to one-inch thickness.
5. Over medium heat in a greased pan (cooking spray), fry each side for approximately 5 minutes.

Calories: 145
Yields: Six patties

Garlic Lemon Tilapia

Ingredients
4 tilapia fillets
1 tablespoon melted butter
3 tablespoons fresh lemon juice
1 finely chopped clove of garlic
1 teaspoon dried parsley flakes

Instructions
1. Set the oven temperature to 375°F. Lightly grease a baking dish.
2. Rinse with cold water and pat dry the fish.
3. Arrange the fillets in the dish with the lemon juice, butter, garlic, pepper and parsley on top.
4. Bake 30 minutes. The fish is done when it is flaky white.

Calories: 142
Yields: Four servings

Marinated Tuna Steak - Grilled

Ingredients

¼ cup each:

- Orange juice
- Soy sauce

1 tbsp. lemon juice

1 clove of garlic - minced

2 tbsp. each:

- Extra-virgin olive oil
- Fresh chopped parsley

½ teaspoons each:

- Ground black pepper
- Chopped fresh oregano

4 (4 ounces) tuna steaks

Instructions

1. Prepare the grill using high heat.
2. Combine the soy sauce, orange juice, lemon juice, olive oil, pepper, garlic, oregano, and parsley in a large dish.
3. Arrange the steaks in the marinade and turn each one to thoroughly coat each piece. Place in a covered dish in the refrigerator for a minimum of 30 minutes.
4. Oil the grill grate and cook the steaks five to six minutes. Flip and baste the other side and cook another five minutes.
5. Discard the marinade.

Calories: 200

Yields: Four servings

Microwave Tilapia

Ingredients
1 pound tilapia fillets
1 minced garlic clove
1 tablespoon butter
¼ cup apple cider vinegar
1 teaspoon fresh chopped tarragon

Instructions
1. Arrange the tilapia in a microwavable dish in a single layer. Add some dotted bits of butter along with the garlic. Sprinkle with the tarragon and cover with a piece of waxed paper.
2. Microwave for two minutes.
3. Flip the fish and continue microwaving for two more minutes on the high setting.
4. Drizzle with the vinegar and enjoy with your favorite side dish.

Calories: 144
Yields: Four servings

Seared Sea Scallops

Ingredients
16 sea scallops – rinsed and drained
½ cup flour - all-purpose
2 teaspoon seasoning salt
2 tbsp. lemon pepper
½ teaspoon each:
- Dried thyme
- Dried oregano
4 teaspoon lemon juice (divided)
4 tbsp. fresh chopped parsley (divided)
2 tbsp. olive oil

1. Whisk the lemon pepper, flour, thyme, oregano, and salt in a mixing bowl. Roll the scallops and cover all sides with the mixture.
2. Warm the oil (high heat) and add four scallops for two minutes per side. Sprinkle with one teaspoon of the juice followed by the parsley. Set them in the oven, and do the same with the remainder of scallops.

Calories: 179
Yields: 4 servings

Steelhead Trout Bake

Ingredients
¼ cup dry white wine
1 pound skinless steelhead trout fillets
1 tbsp. lemon juice
2 ½ tablespoons Dijon mustard
2 pressed garlic cloves
1 teaspoon each:
- Lemon-pepper seasoning
- Dried dill weed

Instructions
1. Lightly spray a baking dish (9x13-inches) with some cooking spray.
2. Program the oven to 400°F.
3. Combine the pepper seasoning, dill, lemon juice, garlic white wine and, mustard in a dish and mix well.
4. Place the fillets in the dish and cover with the sauce.
5. Bake 10 to 15 minutes until the fish easily flakes.

Calories: 145
Yields: Four servings

Szechwan Shrimp

Ingredients
2 teaspoons cornstarch
4 tablespoons water
1 tablespoon each:
- Vegetable oil
- Soy sauce

2 tablespoons ketchup
1 teaspoon honey
4 minced cloves of garlic
¼ teaspoon ground ginger
¼ cup green onions
½ teaspoon crushed red pepper
12 ounces cooked shrimp – no tails

Instructions
1. Mix the ground ginger, red pepper, honey, cornstarch, soy sauce, water, ketchup in a mixing bowl.
2. Warm the oil (medium setting on the stovetop) and blend in the sliced onion and garlic, sautéing for about 30 seconds.
3. Toss in the shrimp with the oil, and empty the sauce in the mix to cook until the sauce is thickened.

Calories: 142 per serving
Yields: Four servings

Other Main Dishes
Zucchini and Tomato Frittata

Ingredients
2 teaspoons olive oil
1 medium diced onion
1-1/2 cups diced zucchini
4 whole large eggs and 4 egg whites

¼ cup Asiago grated cheese

2 medium ripened tomatoes (sliced or crosswise)

Instructions

1. Place the oven setting at 400°F.
2. Add the oil to a 10-inch iron skillet using medium-low temperature.
3. Combine the onion and simmer approximately eight minutes or until browned. Toss in the zucchini with the onions and cook at medium-high.
4. Flavor with salt and pepper if desired. Cook two to three additional minutes or until the moisture is absorbed. Stir occasionally.
5. In the meantime, use another container to whip the eggs, egg whites, and spices. Pour the eggs into the skillet to cover the veggies.
6. Make an arrangement of the eggs overlapping on top of the eggs and cheese. Cook the mixture for about two minutes, and move to the preheated oven for about 15 minutes.

Calories: 172

Yields: Four servings

Sides and Veggies

Beet Pesto Salad

Ingredients

3 beets

¼ cup sesame seeds

2 minced garlic cloves

4 basil leaves

3 tablespoons olive oil

5 ounces feta cheese

Instructions
1. Program the oven temperature to 400°F.
2. Wash and peel the beets and add to some foil with the cloves of garlic. Drizzle **them** with one tablespoon of oil. Wrap tightly and roast one hour. Let the beets cool.
3. In a processor, add two tablespoons of oil, the garlic, seeds, and basil. Blend until creamy smooth.
4. Dice the beets into ½-inch cubes and blend with the pesto and feta cheese in a bowl.
5. Chill for about four hours so the flavors can mingle.

Calories: 88
Yields: 12 servings

Cauliflower and Rice

Ingredients
4 cup cauliflower florets - divided
½ cup or 8 medium chopped green onions
2 tbsp. – divided - olive oil
½ tsp. sea salt flakes
2 tbsp. chopped fresh parsley
1 tbsp. fresh thyme leaves
¼ cup chicken broth - reduced-fat

Instructions
1. With a food processor, add one cup of the cauliflower and coarsely ground until it resembles a grain of rice. Transfer the mixture to a container until all is done. It should make approximately 3 ½ cups of processed product.
2. Use med-high on the stovetop with a skillet, and add one tablespoon of the olive oil. Toss in the onions and salt.
3. Cook for one to two minutes and add the cauliflower along with the remainder of the oil, tossing to cover evenly.

4. Cook for about four to six minutes until the moisture is gone.
5. Add the broth, heating to simmering until the moisture evaporates again, and sprinkle in the thyme and parsley.

Calories: 100
Yields: One serving

Mashed Cauliflower

Ingredients
2 garlic cloves (minced)
1 large head cauliflower
1-ounce chicken broth (low-sodium)
2 tablespoons parmesan cheese (low-sodium)

Instructions
1. Use a steamer and arrange the cauliflower in it until done.
2. In another dish, smash the garlic and cauliflower.
3. Blend in the cheese and broth. Serve hot.

Calories: 66
Yields: Four servings

Potato Salad

Ingredients
1 pound diced potatoes (boiled - steamed)
½ cup each:
- Diced carrot (1 large)
- Diced celery (2 ribs)

1 large (1 cup) yellow onion
2 tbsp. each:
- Minced dill
- Red wine vinegar

1 tsp. black pepper
1/4 cup low-calorie mayonnaise
1 tbsp. Dijon mustard

Instructions
1. Put all of the ingredients in a bowl, combine thoroughly, and enjoy!

Calories: 77 (3/4 cup serving)
Yields: Eight servings

Zucchini Noodles

Ingredients
2 medium zucchini
2 tbsp. olive oil
1 tbsp. black pepper

Instructions
1. Create some long noodles using a potato peeler for each of the zucchini. Continue until you get into the 'gel' part of the zucchini and start the other one.
2. On the stovetop medium-high setting, add the oil and noodles. Saute for two to three minutes.
3. Sprinkle with a bit of pepper and salt and serve with your special pasta sauce.

Calories: 80
Yields: Four servings

Chapter 5: Snacks and Appetizers

The Quick-Fix Snacks

If you are searching for an on-the-go snack, try one of these:

By the Dish:

1 small apple
2 ounces deli turkey
1-ounce sharp cheddar cheese
Calories: 200

1 cup each:
- Chopped cucumber
- Sliced cherry tomatoes

2 tbsp. feta cheese
¼ cup red onion
Accompaniment:
- 2 tbsp. lemon juice
- 1 tsp. olive oil

Calories: 190

½ cup blueberries
Mix with ½ cup each:
- Granola
- Non-fat plain Greek yogurt

Calories: 200

1 cup cherries
¼ cup dark chocolate chips
Calories: 200

½ sliced apple
2 tablespoons lime juice
½ cup each:

- Blueberries
- Strawberries

1 tablespoon raw honey
Calories: 170

½ cup cottage cheese - fat-free
1 cup grilled pineapple
Sprinkle of cinnamon
Calories: 155

1 cup pineapple cubes
2 tablespoons unsweetened coconut flakes
Calories: 175

For Dipping

1 apple
1 tablespoon almond butter
Calories: 170

1 cup sliced strawberries
½ cup non-fat plain Greek frozen yogurt
Calories: 115

¼ cup hummus
½ cup each:
- Baby carrots
- Chopped cucumber
- Sliced red peppers

Calories: 150

Other Combos

1 cup grapes
String cheese
Calories: 140

1 apple
3 cups air-popped popcorn
Calories: 170

1 cup watermelon
Toppings:
- ¼ cup feta cheese
- 1 tsp. fresh chopped dill

Calories: 150

1 hard-boiled egg
½ cup each:
- Sliced cucumber
- Baby carrots
- Sugar snap peas

Dip: 4 tbsp. tzatziki sauce
Calories: 200

Lettuce Wraps:
2 pieces Iceberg lettuce
1 tablespoon mayonnaise
2 ounces deli turkey
2 teaspoons Dijon mustard
Calories: 160

1 small can chicken
Mix with:
- 2 teaspoons Dijon mustard
- 2 tablespoons Greek yogurt

With 1 cup sliced cucumber on the side
Calories: 170

1 baked sweet potato
Sprinkle of cinnamon
½ cup fat-free cottage cheese
Calories: 130

Recipes for Snacks

Bruschetta and Mint Pea Puree

Ingredients
1 French baquette (10 ounces)
2 cloves of garlic
1 package frozen (10 ounces) baby peas
2 tablespoons olive oil
¼ cup fresh mint – finely chopped
1 tablespoon grated Parmesan cheese
3 ounces – room temperature – cream cheese
Pepper and salt

Instructions
1. Set the oven temperature to 375°F.
2. *Prepare the Toast*:
a. Slice the baquette into ½-inch slices (about 30). Bake the slices for 10 minutes.
b. Slice one of the garlic cloves into half.
c. Brush one side of each of the toast pieces with oil and rub with the cut garlic.
d. Return and bake four more minutes and cool.
3. *Make the Puree*:
a. Mince the rest of the clove and combine that along with one-third cup of water and the peas. Cook five minutes after it starts to boil.
b. Puree the mix and let it cool. Toss in the mint and process until blended.
c. When cool, pulse in the parmesan and cream cheese to combine. Add the pepper and salt.
4. *Add to the Toast: Enjoy.*

Calories: 85
Yields: 30 pieces

Jalapeno Fudge

4 fresh chopped jalapenos
3 eggs
16 ounces shredded cheddar cheese
To Taste: Salt and pepper
Butter for the pan

Instructions
1. Warm up the oven to 350°F. Prepare a 9 x 13 baking pan using a small amount of butter.
2. Blend the peppers and eggs and add to the pan. Top with the cheese, pepper, and salt.
3. Bake 30 minutes. Cut and serve warm.

Calories: 86.2 each
Yields: 24 squares

Mexican Jicama Snack

Ingredients
2 juiced limes
1 large jicama
1 tbsp. crushed red pepper

Instructions
1. Peel and slice the jicama into French-fry-sized pieces.
2. Blend the other components. Toss to coat the sticks.
3. Enjoy this as a finger food.

Calories: 84
Yields: Six servings

Sauces

Hummus

Ingredients
¼ cup tahini or 1/3 cup toasted sesame seeds
1 can (15 ounces) garbanzo beans (or 2 cups cooked)
2 tablespoons olive oil
1/8 teaspoon crushed red chilies
½ teaspoon each:
- Minced garlic
- Salt

1/8 cup orange, lemon, or lime juice
1/8 teaspoon crushed red chilies

Instructions
1. Rinse and drain the beans.
2. Heat the oven to 350°F to toast the sesame seeds. Place them on a baking tin and toast them for about eight to twelve minutes. Stir frequently until browned.
3. Use a food processor to puree the chilies, tahini/sesame seeds. Add the beans and continue to puree. Toss in the garlic, salt, and juice of choice. Puree until creamy smooth.
4. Add the oil and continue to process until you reach the desired consistency. To blend the flavors, you need to let the hummus stand for an hour before serving.

Calories: 39
Yields: 1 ½ Cups

Italian Hummus

Ingredients
1 can (15.5 ounces) drained cannellini beans
1 cup non-fat cottage cheese

1 bunch fresh basil
1 pint grape tomatoes
1 minced garlic clove
 Pepper and salt if desired

Instructions
1. Blend all of the ingredients in a blender/food processor until creamy.

Calories: 59
Yields: 12 servings

Orange Basil Vinaigrette

Ingredients
2 tbsp. cornstarch
2 cups orange juice
2 tsp. each:
- Extra-virgin olive oil
- Dried basil (or 1 tbsp. fresh basil)
- Dijon mustard
1/3 cup white wine vinegar

Instructions
1. Using a small pan, mix the cornstarch with the orange juice—bringing it to a boil.
2. Stir constantly, and boil for approximately one minute. Empty the mix into a jar or bowl and place in the refrigerator until well chilled.
3. When chilled and ready to eat, add the vinegar, olive oil, basil, and mustard. Blend until well mixed. Serve right away.

Calories: 45
Yields: Eight servings (1/3 cup each)

Salsa De Tomatillo

Ingredients
1 small chopped onion
10 husked tomatillos
3 chopped garlic cloves
2 chopped jalapeno peppers
¼ cup fresh chopped cilantro
To Taste: Pepper and salt

Instructions
1. Cover the tomatillos with water in a saucepan. Once it boils, simmer about ten minutes (they begin to burst).
2. Drain and add them to a blender/processor along with the remainder of ingredients.
3. Blend until it reaches your chosen consistency.

Calories: 10 calories (1 serving)
Yields: 10 servings

Tzatziki Sauce

Ingredients
2 medium cucumbers
1 garlic clove
3 cup plain yogurt (low-fat)
½ tsp. salt
1 tbsp. fresh chopped dill
3 tbsp. lemon juice
¼ teaspoon black pepper

Instructions
1. Peel and deseed the cucumbers. Add the garlic clove after mincing it.
2. Use a bowl to strain the yogurt using a paper-lined strainer. Put the bowl in the fridge for two hours, so the

yogurt can drain and seep through the strainer. Transfer the strained yogurt into a large bowl.

3. In a small mixing dish, grate the cucumber—sprinkling with the salt.
4. Wrap the cucumber in towels to remove the liquid and add it to the yogurt.
5. Blend in the garlic kill, lemon juice, pepper, and the remainder of the salt.
6. Let the sauce blend in the refrigerator for several hours.
7. Serve chilled or at room temperature.

Calories: 37 (¼ cup servings)
Yields: 3 ½ Cups

Vegetable Salsa

Ingredients
2 green bell peppers (approx. 2 cups)
1 cup chopped red onion
2 red bell green peppers (about 2 cups)
1 cup diced zucchini
4 diced tomatoes (approx. 2 cups)
½ cup chopped fresh cilantro
½ tsp. salt
2 minced garlic cloves
1 tsp. ground black pepper
2 tsp. sugar
¼ cup lime juice

Instructions
1. Prepare all of the vegetables by washing them completely. Seed and dice the peppers and the tomatoes. Chop the zucchini, red onion, and cilantro. Mince the garlic.

2. Toss all of the listed ingredients into a container, stir, and cover. Let the salsa rest in the fridge for a minimum of thirty minutes for the ingredients to blend.

Calories: 24
Yields: 16 servings

Chapter 6: Desserts

Apples and Cream Cheese Roll-Ups

Ingredients for the Filling
1/3 cup apple juice concentrate (undiluted and thawed)
1 cup chopped dried apples
Dash of ground nutmeg
¼ teaspoon ground cinnamon
¼ cup each:
- (2 ounces) low-fat cream cheese
- Sugar

1 large egg

Ingredients for the Pastry
Cooking spray
12 sheets frozen phyllo/filo dough (thawed)
½ cup – divided - graham cracker crumbs

Ingredients for the Topping
½ teaspoon cinnamon
1 ½ teaspoons sugar

Instructions
1. Program the oven to 350°F. Spray some spray cooking oil on a baking tin.
2. *Make the Filling*: Use the med-high setting and combine the apples, concentrate, cinnamon, and nutmeg. When it boils, cover, and lower the temperature to simmer for five minutes.
3. Cool (room temperature), and blend in the cream cheese and sugar using a mixer using the lowest speed. Add the egg and blend. Combine with the apple mixture.
4. *Prepare the Pastry*: Arrange the pastry on the countertop and coat with the cooking spray. Sprinkle it using one teaspoon sugar and two teaspoons of the crumbs.

5. Cut the phyllo stack into six strips, and spoon a rounded teaspoon of the apples approximately ½ inch from the end of the strip. Roll them up arranging seam sides on the baking sheet.
6. *Make the Topping*: Combine the ingredients and spread them over the rolls.
7. Bake for ten minutes and cool on a wire rack.

Calories: 81 (1 roll up)
Yields: 24 servings

Banana Bread (Whole Grain)

Ingredients
¾ cup egg whites/egg substitute
½ cup each:
- Quinoa flour
- Millet flour
- Rice flour
- Tapioca flour
- Amaranth flour brown

1 teaspoon baking soda
1/8 teaspoon salt
2 tablespoons grape seed oil
2 cups mashed banana
½ cup raw sugar

Instructions
1. Prepare a loaf pan (5 x 9) with a dusting of cooking spray. Sprinkle with some flour and set to the side.
2. Preheat the oven setting to 350°F.
3. Mix all of the dry ingredients—omitting the sugar—in a large bowl.
4. In another dish, blend the egg, oil, mashed banana, and sugar.

5. Blend all of the ingredients and thoroughly mix, adding them to the loaf pan.
6. Bake for 50 to 60 minutes. Cool, slice, and enjoy.

Calories: 150
Yields: Serves 14

Blueberry Shortbread Bites

Ingredients
2/3 cup sugar
1-½ cups flour
¼ cup cornstarch
¼ teaspoon salt
1 tablespoon orange zest (finely shredded)
2/3 cup dried blueberries
¾ cup cubed cold butter
Also Need: Food Processor

Instructions
1. Program the oven to 350°F. Prepare 36 mini muffin cups.
2. Pulse the zest, salt, cornstarch, sugar, flour. Toss in the butter. Pulse until it is crumbly fine. Remove the dish and blend in the berries.
3. Scoop out 2 tablespoons of the batter and press firmly into the cups.
4. Bake about 15 minutes and cool before serving. For regular muffins, you can use ¼ cup mixture into 18 cups for 20 minutes (adjust the calories).

Calories: 82 each
Yields: 36 bites

Coconut Chocolate Cookies

Ingredients
1 cup each:
- Flaked sweetened coconut
- All-purpose flour

¼ tsp. baking soda
¾ cup packed brown sugar
1/8 tsp. salt
½ tsp. baking powder
1 large egg
¼ cup softened unsalted butter
2 ounces chopped dark chocolate (70% cacao)
1 teaspoon vanilla extract

Instructions
1. Prepare the oven to 350°F.
2. In a small baking pan, arrange the coconut, and bake for 7 minutes (stir once). Remove and let it cool.
3. Combine and mix the salt, flour, and baking soda and powder in a mixing dish.
4. Empty the sugar and butter into a separate container and blend on the medium speed using a mixer. Blend in the egg and vanilla. Pour in the flour and beat until slightly combined. Add the chocolate and coconut.
5. Drop the cookies about two inches apart (one tablespoon leveled), and bake for ten minutes. Cool on wire racks.

Calories: 88 (1 cookie)
Yields: 25 Servings

Ginger Snap Cookies

Ingredients
1 large egg
¼ cup unsalted butter
1 teaspoon vanilla extract
1 cup sugar substitute/Erythritol (Swerve)
½ teaspoon ground cinnamon
2 teaspoons ground ginger
2 cups almond flour
¼ teaspoon each:
- Salt
- Ground cloves
- Nutmeg

Instructions
1. Set the oven to 350°F.
2. Mix all of the dry ingredients in a small dish.
3. Blend the remainder of the components to the dry mixture, and mix using a hand blender/mixer. (The dough will be crumbly and stiff.)
4. Measure out the dough for each cookie and flatten with a fork or your fingers. Bake for approximately 9 to 11 minutes or till they are browned.

Calories: 74 (1 cookie per serving)
Yields: 24 cookies

Simmered Pears

Ingredients
¼ cup apple juice
1 cup orange juice
1 teaspoon each:
- Ground nutmeg
- Cinnamon
½ cup fresh raspberries
4 whole pears

2 tablespoons orange zest

Instructions
1. Peel the pears leaving the stems on. Use a coring tool to remove the core from the bottom/base. Put in a shallow baking dish.
2. Over medium heat, blend the juices, nutmeg, and cinnamon, stirring until evenly mixed.
3. Do not boil, but simmer for thirty minutes, turning the pears often.
4. Take them from the dish; garnish with the orange zest and raspberries.

Calories: 140 (1 pear)
Yields: Four Servings

Very Berry Tarts

Ingredients
½ teaspoon grated lemon rind
1 cup vanilla low-fat yogurt
½ cup each:
- Frozen fat-free whipped topping (thawed)
- ½ cup (+) 2 tablespoons *Triple Berry Curd* (see recipe)

2 (2.1 ounces) package mini phyllo shells (I used Athens)
Optional Garnish: Grated lemon rind

Instructions
1. Scoop out the yogurt onto paper plates/towels to absorb extra moisture while spreading it out to ½-inch thickness. Cover for five minutes and add to a mixing dish.
2. Blend the lemon rind and yogurt. Fold in the whipped topping.
3. Spoon one teaspoon of the *Triple Berry Curd* (below) into each shell followed by 2 teaspoons of the yogurt mix.

4. Garnish and serve immediately

Calories: 63 (2 tarts each serving)
Yields: 15 servings

Triple Berry Curd

Ingredients
1 cup each frozen and thawed:
- Raspberries
- Blueberries
- Blackberries

1/8 tsp. salt
1 tbsp. cornstarch
3 large eggs
2/3 cup sugar
2 tbsp. each:
- Butter
- Fresh lemon juice

Instructions
1. Process the berries in a blender until smooth. Press the ingredients through a sieve to reserve one cup of puree.
2. In a heavy saucepan (med. heat), mix the salt, cornstarch, and sugar. Whisk the juice, eggs, and one cup of puree.
3. When the mixture begins to boil, lower the temperature and simmer one minute.
4. Remove it from the burner, and add the butter.
5. Cool and spoon the curd into a covered dish and chill for a minimum of six hours. Overnight is best since it thickens as it cools.

Calories: 29 (1 tablespoon per serving)
Yields: 2 ½ cups

Conclusion

Thank for making it through to the end of your personal copy of the *Lose Your Belly Diet*. Let's hope it was informative and provided you with all of the tools you need to achieve your goals of weight gain or loss.

The next step is to set your game plan in motion. This is what you have learned to keep you in line and healthier:

What to Eat

- *Fresh, Canned, or Frozen Veggies*
- *Frozen, Fresh, or Canned Fruits*
- *Calcium-Rich Foods*
- *Alter the Methods of Cooking*

Stay Focused!

How to Snack Healthy

- *Always read the food panels.*
- *Use pre-packaged snack packs.*
- *Remove the temptations.*
- *Plan ahead.*
- *Choose fiber food items.*

Finally, if you found this book useful in any way, a review on Amazon is always appreciated!